Also by James Occhiogrosso

Solutions for Erectile Dysfunction
Your Prostate, Your Libido, Your Life
Dr. Jim's Guide to the Aging Male Body

Watch for more at www.prostatehealthnaturally.com/index.html.

Dr. Jim's Guide to the Aging Male Body

James Occhiogrosso, N.D.

A Guide to Understanding and Minimizing Aging Effects on Men.

Introduction

C ongratulations. By reading this book you are opening yourself up to a wealth of information that you will not get from your friends at the gym or your doctor. As an aged man and practicing health professional for many years, I have come across just about every problem that plagues men as they age beyond fifty and into their nineties.

Over the years, I have seen several thousand clients, most of them aging men. In many cases, I sympathize with them since – at various times in my life – I have joined in their suffering with similar aging male problems. As I write this, I am a happily married man approaching my 82nd birthday. Much of what I say in this book is based on my observations of the problems and solutions of many of my both myself and many of my clients.

As men age, especially after they turn fifty, they often encounter problems they never knew before, many of them sexual. Facing symptoms such as; loss of interest in sex, erectile dysfunction, and urinary issues, they are prime targets for a wealth of charlatans that simply want to dip into their wallets and help themselves to the contents.

These charlatans come in many flavors, from the late night TV ads for ED, to the urologist that recommends surgical prostate removal based on a PSA test with a single out-of-range result. Many of my clients have had surgery that was unwarranted, mostly in the form of prostate surgery. A recent study in the New England Journal of Medicine suggested that close to 80 percent of prostate surgery was unwarranted.

You will likely find that this book contradicts things you have learned from other sources, particularly the media and maybe even some of the health professionals you have visited. Be advised though, that the information contained herein, is either from my own experience or practice, my discussions of similar experiences with other health providers, or from scientific studies produced by reputable scientists.

Much of what is circulated today comes from myths perpetuated by the media, pharmaceutical companies, or shady medical practices. For years, male aging issues and advertisements for male enhancement products and testosterone supplementation have been ubiquitous in the media.

"Low-T" has fast become a well-known term and many men have come to believe the myth that most or all of their aging problems can be fixed simply with a visit to a doctor and a prescription for testosterone.

- *Myth-buster:* **While low testosterone might result in a flagging libido, it is usually not the primary cause of ED.**

This universal oversimplification of a very complex issue has led many men to disaster. While testosterone is indeed an extremely important hormone for a man, it is but one instrument in a very complex orchestra, and, excess testosterone levels can be dangerous to your health.

This book is about learning what is real and will work verses the myths perpetuated by various websites and merchants simply looking to use your problems to part you from your money.

In some instances, you will find items in this book in direct contradiction of what you think you already know or have been told by friends or a medical professional. If this occurs, I suggest you research the item carefully and decide for yourself what is real and what is myth or hype.

My goal in writing this is not to sell you anything other than the knowledge contained in this book, all of it well researched and proven by actual trial and experience. I have generally tried to avoid recommendations for treatment of any condition

I do mention a few natural supplements or herbals that are known to help certain conditions, but, I caution the reader that these are mentioned simply to provide a starting point for your own additional research.

Natural products often require specific dosing and extraction techniques to do their job, but some supplement manufacturers throw products together based on marketing information rather than efficacy. The solution is either to do your own extensive research or partner with a natural health provider who is knowledgeable in treating your condition.

The topics in this book are not in order or importance, since the level of concern is different with everyone. Instead, they are in alphabetical order.

Certain topics already have a wealth of published information about them, and a chapter in this book would simply be very redundant. However, there are some topics, such as, erectile dysfunction and prostate cancer, where charlatans or misinformation are prevalent or I have written extensively about it elsewhere.

For example: The topic of erectile dysfunction has just a cursory overview in this book, since I already have an extensive book available at all major booksellers on that subject called "Solutions for Erectile Dysfunction".

Prostate cancer (PC) is also a topic with a wealth of information about it currently available elsewhere. My book "Your Prostate, Your Libido, Your Life", provides many natural ways to improve your overall health and the health of your prostate. While it was published more than ten years ago, most of the information in it is stilll quite relevent today.

The chapter in this book is more about avoiding a disaster if you get a PC diagnosis sometime in your life.

Caution: – Throughout this book, I have placed bolded caution markers where unscrupulous medical personnel have seized on minor problems of their clients and led them into more comprehensive and aggressive treatments. Generally, this involved implementing a treatment or medical procedure that was not really justified.

Many of these cases actually caused harm to the patient, often in the form of unanticipated side effects never mentioned by the medical practitioner. In some cases, these unneeded procedures caused nothing more than temporary discomfort. Other cases carried some permanent unwanted side effects, and in one case the outcome was fatal.

The "About the Author" page of this book contains contact information for me, and I will, to the best of my ability answer all email. However, while I can point you in a direction that might help with a problem, I cannot attempt to diagnose specific problems.

It is my sincere hope that this book will help you understand some of the problems you might face as you age gracefully, and make you better able to rectify them, and I will be happy to hear from you in that regard.

Diet and Lifestyle

Many of the problems encountered as as man ages can be improved with a judicious approach to improving overall health by improving ones diet and lifestyle.

One of the biggest health issues in the US is obesity. Statistics indicate that nearly 40 percent of adult men in the US are obese, and more than 30 percent are overweight but not yet obese. In all, more than two-thirds of adults in the United States carry to much weight.

Hundreds of studies support obesity as a risk factor for cancer, cardiac problems and other health conditions, both serious and minor.

Obesity is known to alter endocrine status, increase oxidative stress and contribute to an increased systemic inflammation process. Lifestyle issues, such as poor diet, lack of exercise, stress, and other issues that promote systemic inflammation are also contributors.

Diabetes is a disease that has well-known ties to diet and obesity. It is also well known that it is associated with ED and BPH, both of which are common in older men. Obese men with high blood sugar levels also seem to have a high risk of chronic prostatitis.

Aging does not specifically initiate disease! It is the association of aging with poor diet and lifestyle that initiates most health problems. A young body can handle many health insults readily, but it is a whole different story, when the same health insults impact a body 20, 30, or 50 years older.

An aging man that is encountering almost any of the issues in this book should take a hard look at his diet and lifestyle and take steps to decrease his inflammatory loading and improve his overall health.

A bulging belly might be the source of jovial commentary, but the fun ceases when your sex life crashes, you are gasping for breath on minor exertion, or lying in a hospital bed with tubes coming out of everywhere.

Common Male Aging Problems

There are many changes that occur in the human body as we age. For women, many are due to general aging or associated with the cessation of menstrual flow (menopause) that occurs around the age of 50. Men do not have a specific marker to refer to, but the changes are there nevertheless.

There is no specific order or age when one of these problems may appear in a man's life, so I have identified each of the problems by its common name and put them in separate chapters ordered alphabetically to aid in navigation thru the book.

Some men – the really lucky ones – will see few, if any, of these issues, and others will see multiple issues. With the exception of prostate cancer, the issues I talk about in this book are not diseases. Some such as, prostatitis are relatively common, others like anorgasmia, relatively rare.

Almost all are correctable with natural techniques and a few might need some medical intervention. However, if you have a choice, keep in mind that natural techniques carry few undesired side effects, while medical treatment might solve one problem and create one or more problems elsewhere.

My goal with this book is to educate you about the types of problems you might encounter as you age so that you are aware of them. Treatment for a particular condition may differ from person to person depending on individual circumstances, thus there are no treatment recommendations in this book.

My advice is that if you have one of conditions listed, learn about the basics of the condition from this book, then seek more complete

Testing a man's prolactin level is requires only a simple and inexpensive blood test.

Anorgasmia or orgasmic dysfunction is also prevalent among diabetic men. This is likely due to nerve desensitization, similar to the peripheral neuropathy that often affects peripheral nerves in the hands and feet of diabetic men.

To the best of my knowledge, there are no drugs or herbal remedies that directly affect anorgasmia, and few doctors are knowledgeable about the condition. Dietary and lifestyle changes might help, particularly those that reduce obesity and help control diabetes.

Benign Prostate Enlargement (BPH)

———

B enign Prostate Enlargement or BPH is likely the most common problem encountered by the aging male. It is a nonmalignant enlargement of the prostate gland beyond its normal size. Typically, this growth begins in a man's fifties and continues as he gets older.

Initially, it causes few symptoms other than a gradual slowdown in urinary voiding. While the causes of BPH are not specifically identified, most men with serious issues tend to be overweight and heavy consumers of the Standard American Diet (otherwise known as SAD!)

In some families, it is common among the male members, indicating that it may have a strong genetic component.

- *Myth-Buster: BPH does not lead to or cause Prostate Cancer. However, the two conditions sometimes exist in the same person.*

Since the male prostate surrounds the tube that allows urine to pass from the urinary bladder through the penis (the urethra) the age-related excess growth associated with BPH can often compromise prostate or urinary function and treatment – either natural or medical treatment may be required.

Symptoms typically include a frequent need or urgency to urinate, difficulty in starting or stopping urination, urine leakage, a weak, interrupted or split urine stream, blood in the urine, inability to void completely (urinary retention), and interruption of normal sleep due to the need to urinate (nocturia).

Symptoms can also include erectile or orgasm problems. The most serious problem is when the prostate growth interferes substantially with normal urinary flow. In severe cases, the flow of urine can be totally blocked, which is a medical emergency requiring immediate medical intervention.

Typically, men with symptoms of BPH are given prescription medication, but studies show that a properly formulated herbal supplement can be just as effective for most men. Prescription medication may solve the immediate problem, but does little to correct the cause, and often causes unpleasant side effects.

Conventional Medical Treatments for BPH – Medical treatments for BPH typically use the drugs, Finasteride (Proscar, Propecia), Dutasteride (Avodart, Duogen), or Tamsulosin (Flomax). Each has significant side effects including loss of libido, pain on ejaculation, inability to have an orgasm, erectile dysfunction, dizziness, vision problems, and excess breast growth.

Recent studies indicate that Finasteride can reduce the risk of prostate cancer, however, the prevention aspect is dulled by the under-reported detail that it also appears to increase risk of developing aggressive and potentially fatal prostate cancer.

Mnay urologists also offer surgical treatments for BPH. The most common of which is called a Transurethral Resection of the Prostate (TURP). This treatment is what many men refer to as a "roto-rooter-job" after the company that cleans clogged household plumbing.

The above analogy is pretty accurate, since the TURP procedure essentially removes the excess prostate growth into the urethra by either cutting or burning it away.

Herbal Products that can Resolve BPH Symptoms – While there are many herbal supplements being sold today to help rectify problems associated with BPH, the four items listed below have a significant amount of scientific studies proving their value. Synergy is a term used by herbalists. It indicates a combination of herbal ingredients can work together to significantly increase the effectiveness of a properly formulated combination product. Thus, such products can be more effective than a drug and can often help resolve some sexual issues as well as helping with prostate enlargement.

Saw palmetto, pygeum, nettle, and pumpkin seed oil all have slightly different effects on the prostate and can work together in a synergistic relationship to provide multiple beneficial effects. There is strong evidence that the synergistic effect of such combinations—can significantly improve prostate health and reduce symptoms of BPH when used regularly.

Saw Palmetto (Serenoa repens) – In Europe, saw palmetto is the primary choice for treatment for BPH. It has also shown value in treating erectile dysfunction. Saw palmetto has a long history of use for prostate problems, particularly BPH, and is known to be quite safe. In recent European studies, it provided significant improvement in maximum urinary flow, a decrease in overall prostate size, and improvement in other symptoms including sexual function. However, while symptom improvements were noted within a month of starting treatment, the maximum benefits were not evident until after a year or so. This suggests that treatment with saw palmetto may initiate a long-term healing process within the prostate.

Saw palmetto has very few side effects, and many men report that it enhances libido and erectile function. It is quite possible however, that the reduction in prostate size and the improvement of overall urinary health could result in a feeling of well being that could easily account for the increased sexual performance.

Some supplement manufacturers sell ground saw palmetto berries in capsules. While the berries are indeed healthy, to see significant improvement in prostate problems you would need to swallow a significant number of capsules. With many herbal remedies, only a concentrated and standardized extract is effective—and, such extracts are expensive—hence the reason why some inexpensive supplements do nothing. While saw palmetto extract is effective by itself, it is even more effective when used along with other herbs, like pygeum, nettle, and pumpkin seed oil (described below) for the synergistic effect.

Pygeum (Pygeum africanum, Prunus africana) – Pygeum bark is traditionally used with saw palmetto for the treatment of urinary and prostate problems. A recent analysis that looked at eighteen, controlled trials including a total of 1562 men with BPH concluded that pygeum improves the urinary symptoms with few side effects. Significant improvements were noted in nighttime voiding, urinary flow and volume, all persistently annoying symptoms of BPH. Other studies have indicated that, like saw palmetto, the full effects of supplementing with pygeum are only obtained using a properly formulated extract over a long period of regular use.

Stinging Nettle Root (Urtica dioica) – Stinging nettle (or simply nettle) is a weed-like plant that grows wild throughout the United States. It has a long history of therapeutic use for many different health issues. Both the root and the leaves of the plant are used medicinally. Nettle root is effective for treating BPH. Like saw palmetto and pygeum, nettle contains many phytosterols that can help relieve symptoms of prostate dysfunction.

By itself, nettle it is not quite as effective as saw palmetto or pygeum in treating BPH, but since it operates slightly differently, it is usually combined with both for the synergistic effect. Several studies conclude that the plant sterols in nettle root inhibited activity of certain prostate cells in such a way as to help prevent the excess growth of BPH, and possibly slow the growth of prostate cancer. In animals induced in the laboratory to have four times the normal prostate tissue, nettle reduced the excess tissue by more than one-third. In addition, nettle has anti-inflammatory properties that make it effective for treating chronic prostatitis.

Pumpkin (Cucurbita pepo) Seed Oil – Pumpkin Seed Oil contains high amounts of omega-3 essential fatty acids, protein, amino acids, iron, phosphorous, and zinc—all of which have significant value for prostate health. Historically, pumpkin seeds have been used in many cultures, including Native Americans, to treat BPH and prostatitis. There is evidence that they may also help control prostate cancer. In a study of fifty-three men with BPH, urinary flow, residual urine, urgency and frequency of urination were significantly improved. Many European countries have formally approved pumpkin seeds and pumpkin seed oil for the treatment of BPH.

Erectile Dysfunction

Unfortunately, ED, like many other health conditions, can be caused by chronic nutrient deficiencies that have been perpetuated for many years. Contrary to what the pharmaceutical industry would have you believe, it is not a simple problem, easily fixed with a drug, but a complex chronic disorder involving several body systems. And, it is often an indicator of a more serious underlying disease.

Physicians sometimes mislead patients. Not because they mean to, but because they tend to treat symptoms instead of resolving the underlying problems that cause them. Treating symptoms of a chronic condition can make the patient feel better. But without a coherent, long-term approach towards correcting the underlying cause, treating symptoms does little for a patient's overall prognosis. And in certain cases, treating and suppressing symptoms may actually do more harm than good.

Erectile Dysfunction is a good example of the above. The male penis is essentially a plumbing device. When a man is aroused, a complex process occurs between the brain and the body that results in signals that cause arteries to open, fill the penis with blood and become erect.

Clogged arteries will prevent this from happening. Generally, the body does not single out penile arteries and specifically clog them. Thus, when a man encounters ED, it is often due to obstruction of blood flow, which is, in turn, due either to generally poor circulation or obstruction of arteries throughout the body.

Men do no generally understand the relationship between ED and the cardiovascular system. While ED does not specifically indicate a man has a circulation issue, it may be the first symptom of a underlying cardiac or circulatory condition.

Most men have few problems with erectile dysfunction in their youth and expect such youthful vigor to continue forever. However, as the years advance, the health and vitality of the body deteriorates, and the level of sexual vigor drops accordingly. Unfortunately, many men that suffer from erectile dysfunction, loss of libido, or both, cannot (or will not) admit to a connection between their problems and their overall health.

Most cases of erectile dysfunction are due to impaired blood circulation resulting from an underlying health condition. An organ lacking good blood circulation cannot maintain peak health. The penis is no exception. The overall health of the penis is dependent on good blood circulation. It needs an ample blood supply for nourishment and general tissue health. Thus, erectile dysfunction can be the first symptom of compromised vascular system, and is often an early symptom of other cardiovascular problems.

Any health condition, medication, or physical injury that impedes blood circulation in a man often results in some degree of erectile dysfunction. To produce an erection for sexual activity requires an unimpeded blood circulation to the penis. Thus, while some cases of erectile dysfunction are related to hormone imbalances, the problem is more often a direct result of poor health or vascular insufficiency.

Men that encounter ED that has no obvious cause should be screened for cardiovascular disease even if they have no other symptoms. Unfortunately, this is not the norm. Many doctors simply write a prescription for one of the ED medications, and the guy goes on his merry way – at least until his sexual activity is interrupted by a heart attack!

My book, "Your Prostate, Your Libido, Your Life" contains extensive information of the causes of ED. If you already know the cause, my book "Solutions for Erectile Dysfunction" offers many ways to overcome specific types of ED. Both are available at book selling sites on-line and in book stores.

Erectile dysfunction is common among men of all ages and particularly in older men. It can sometimes by easily rectified with a drug or an herbal remedy. However, it is important for any man that has consistent problems getting or keeping an erection, to consult with an expert that deals with the problem regularly.

Loss of Libido

———

L ibido is a word that refers to sexual desire or drive. While many men mistakenly believe that low testosterone is the primary cause of ED, it typically has little actual effect on a man's erection. However, low testosterone typically results in little desire or no desire for sexual activity (low libido). The connection to ED is more associated with the low drive, than with an actual erectile problem. If one has no desire for sex, it is also likely that one will have problems attaining an erection.

Libido for both a man or a woman is controlled by a combination of hormones and processes in the body. It is a complex combination of physical conditions, hormonal balance, nerve function, circulatory and overall health, as well as external stimuli to the brain. Anything that interferes with any of these pathways can cause a problem. Low libido is often a side effect of medical treatments and/or medications.

People vary considerable in their need for sexual activity. There are those that are quite content with rare or non-existent sexual activity as well as those that that are unhappy if they do not have sexual activity on a daily or near daily basis. There is no normal level and libido cannot be measured in a laboratory. What is normal for one person, may be way out of range for another.

Problems typically occur when two people in a sexual relationship have vastly different libido levels. This often results in serious emotional problems and is likely the unmentioned source of marital incompatibilities and many divorces.

Medications, especially antidepressants, can cause or exacerbate a loss of libido. Thus, an unwary man can easily become trapped in a vicious cycle.

A low testosterone level might cause depression, for which treatment is attempted with various antidepressant medication.

If his depression is treated with antidepressants, his libido may decrease even more, and he then may experience medication-related erectile dysfunction, further increasing his depression and compounding his problems. The Association for Male Sexual Dysfunction recognizes over 200 drugs that may affect sexual performance.

Low libido can also be caused by various medications for treating blood pressure and other medical conditions. If you have had a low libido level throughout life, it is likely that is your set point. There is little you can do to change it. If however, you have a sudden decrease in libido, especially if coupled with the onset of a new medication, I recommend you research that medication and its side effects. Sometimes a change in medication can resolve the issue.

Low libido can also be associated with an underlying medical condition. Be aware though, diagnosing such problems is often impossible for a medical practitioner and self-diagnosis might be the only way to get a handle on the cause.

Nocturnal Erections

The male body has a built-in testosterone measuring system that most men are very unaware of. Young men usually have regular erections during sleep, typically in the early morning hours. Some will wake and notice the erection, others may be barely aware of it, but this action is the body's way of exercising the male anatomy and keeping it healthy.

This process is highly dependent on testosterone level. When a man has a normal testosterone level he will typically have an erection almost every day in the early morning hours. This erection is not based on sexual arousal, although it may be accompanied by an erotic dream. But, it is simply the bodies way of exercising the mechanism.

In the section above on ED, I talk about the myth perpetuated on men about how testosterone is what counts for a guy to get an erection. Testosterone is a major player for the health of many body systems, but low levels are not the main cause of ED.

Adequate testosterone levels are essential for a man to have normal libido, orgasms, and spontaneous erections. Unfortunately, there is no specific value to determine what an adequate or normal level is. What is normal for one man may be woefully insufficient for another. If your testosterone levels fall on the low side of the normal range and you are having symptoms of low testosterone, replacement therapy may be in order, particularly if you are not experiencing nocturnal erections.

If you do have very low levels, it is advisable to see your doctor before doing anything natural. Low testosterone levels can be caused by a benign pituitary tumor or other conditions, and it is wise to rule these out first. If your levels are very low, and all medical causes are ruled out,

our doctor can prescribe a bio-identical transdermal testosterone cream
or you.

There appears to be two distinct chemical paths to spontaneous
nocturnal erections. The first is highly dependent on testosterone and
he second dependent on nerve communication and other chemical
ignaling. Men with low free testosterone levels generally have missing
or significantly less powerful nocturnal erections than men with normal
evels. However, testosterone levels do not appear to directly effect
rections induced by other erotic stimuli.

Thus, while testosterone level is extremely important, it is but one player
n this complex orchestra. If you are having sexual difficulties, and you
re not experiencing spontaneous nocturnal or early morning erections,
ou should have both your total and free testosterone levels checked. See
he Testosterone section below for specific levels.

Penile Shrinkage

The thought of your penis shrinking may bring you nervous anxiet and chill-bumps. However, it is very normal for a man to lose little size (mostly in length) with aging. With aging, some deposits of fa and plaque are inevitable and they do cause a reduction of oxyge carrying blood to the penis, thus weakening muscles cells within th penis that are involved in an erection.

Any loss in size is generally important to a man only on the erect peni There is little mention of penile shrinkage in the flaccid penis in variou studies I have reviewed. For a healthy man, the effect is relatively sma (usually only about a centimeter or less), and often goes unnotice However, there are several conditions that may cause a greater loss. Thes are:

- Prostate or Pelvic surgery, particularly a prostatectomy or a TURP.
- Long-term low testosterone levels.
- Long periods of little to no sexual activity.

Any of the above can cause significant reduction in both flaccid an erect penile length. For guys that have had surgery, drugs in the EI family of PDE5 inhibitors, if started early after surgery, can help reduc size loss but only if some sexual activity is maintained. Many urologist that perform these surgeries start their patients on a PDE5 inhibito immediately after surgery to help regain sexual activity as soon a possible as well as prevent penile shrinkage.

In my years of practice, I have seen many men with severely reduced peni size. A normal penis is typically a little under six inches when erect. A few men have indicated that their size was normal when younger, but had shrunken by more than an inch (erect length) over time. One of them had an erect length of less than 5 cm (about 2 inches).

On further examination and detailed history, each of these men admitted to a long-term lack of sexual activity. In three cases the lack of activity was more than ten years. Activity was defined as sexual arousal of any kind, including masturbation or pornography. Each of these guys reported a a lack of nocturnal erections as well.

One of them in particular, was now into a relationship with a woman that was highly desirous of sex. He was in his early 60's and had not had any kind of sexual activity for about 12 years,. He did have a relatively normal sex life before he voluntarily went celibate, and he was highly motivated to resume sexual activity with his new partner. However, no matter what I recommended, there was little to no improvement. Even the use of direct penile injections, provided little improvement. He eventually went to a surgeon and had a penile prosthesis implanted.

A penile prosthesis is where the internal chambers of the penis are replaced by rubber tubes that are inflated with a saline solution from a reservoir embedded in the scrotum. While it may look natural cosmetically, I have yet to meet a man that prefers it over the original!

The other two cases were similar. But neither man was highly motivated. Both expected immediate results, and when that was not the case, gave up trying shortly thereafter. To the best of my knowledge, neither regained any ability to have a normal sex life.

As a natural health practitioner, I have found that many men are very impatient regarding this sort of issue. While their size loss most likely occurred over a span of 10 or more years, they expect a remedy quickly and lose interest if they do not get results in a short time.

The reality is that if a loss took ten or more years to happen, there is little hope for a quick recovery. In many cases, recovery may not be possible, ever! Think about tying your arm to the side of your body and not using it for ten years or so. Muscles that are not used tend to weaken and become unusable. The medical term for this is atrophy, and it applies equally well to your unused penis as it does to your tied up arm! The bottom line is – use it or lose it!

Some men find they are in a situation where sexual activity is non-existent or impossible. This often occurs after a long-time married man loses a spouse or there is a divorce. If you are in this situation, you need to take steps to avoid atrophy of your penis or the nerve connections to it. There are several ways to accomplish this as follows:

- Purchase a vacuum erection device (AKA: penis pump) and use it daily. Mornings are best to mimic the natural state of early morning or nocturnal erections. A penis pump simulates an erection by applying a vacuum to the penis. This draws blood into the penis causing an erection. It is not as good as the real thing, but it does help prevent atrophy.
- Masturbate regularly.
- Find a sexual partner.

Remember, it is far easier to prevent penile shrinkage than it is to recover from it.

Prostate Cancer

———

Most men are highly concerned about prostate cancer, and it has become a media hot button. However, prostate cancer comes in many varieties, most of which are very slow-growing and non-aggressive and may never become a threat to life or one's sexual health.

Every case of prostate cancer has multiple varied treatment options, including indolent type of cancer that may need little to no treatment other than long-term monitoring. Much information is available in the form of books, websites and articles that deal with prostate cancer, thus I will not discuss the multiple treatment options and their ramifications here.

Instead, I will discuss the typical scenarios that lead a man into the serious medical nightmare that is prostate cancer, which will often leave him a sexual cripple for life.

A good source for learning more about prostate cancer is the book "Invasion of the Prostate Snatchers" by Mark Scholz, MD and and Ralph H. Blum, available at book sellers everywhere. I highly recommend this book for any man that is concerned about prostate cancer.

Almost every article you will read about prostate cancer begins with statistical information about how many cases are diagnosed yearly and how many men die from it. Also, the bulk of the written documentation refers to and details various treatment modalities.

According to the American Cancer Society, prostate cancer is the most frequently diagnosed cancer in men. Each year, more than 220,000 cases are diagnosed, and approximately 27,000 of them eventually result in death due to the disease. For most men, such a diagnosis is devastating, representing their worst fears.

Statistics like these—frequently cited in mainstream news media—certainly add to the apprehension every man feels as the time for his annual physical rolls around. But what these statistics do not show is that many newly diagnosed cases of prostate cancer are low risk and may not need immediate treatment.

Also the statistics might be misleading. The father of a friend of mine died at the tender age of 93. His death was attributed to prostate cancer. Now, while his record surely contained his prostate cancer diagnosis, that condition had been diagnosed more than 20 years earlier. In my opinion, it is very likely that his prostate cancer was of an indolent type and his death more likely due to some organ failure from advanced age. But, prostate cancer was on his record and I would be willing to bet that his death was added to the prostate cancers statistics.

How many doctors have the time to spend detailing the exact cause of a hospitalized 93 YO man's death? Being that no autopsy was to be performed Perhaps, the easy answer was to choose the "known" illness for the death certificate.

What most men are not aware of, and what is *not* "up front" in the media reports, is that prostate cancer is usually slow growing and that men with low or favorable risk cancer may *never* need aggressive treatment.

A man might have undiagnosed prostate cancer for years without even being aware of it. Autopsies of men who died from various causes have consistently shown that undiagnosed prostate cancer is common. It is estimated that about 40 percent of men in their fifties to about 80 percent of men in their seventies have latent or undiagnosed prostate cancer.

t is also estimated (from autopsy studies) that the rate of indolent prostate cancer in older men is about equal to their age in percentage. ndolent prostate cancer has a high probability of never causing clinical disease. This results in overdiagnosis,and because many are treated to nsure that all cancers are treated, overtreatment.

n a recent article in *PCRI Insights,* Dr. Laurence Klotz of the University of Toronto states, "50-60% of diagnosed patients now fall into the favorable-risk category." Unfortunately, many of these low-risk patients will still receive immediate aggressive treatment that they may not really need.

The side effects of almost every kind of treatment are often a complete oss of normal sexual function. Some doctors that perform such procedures are in denial about this!

Fear of dying from cancer is a strong motivator and some practitioners stoke that fear with dire predictions of doom and gloom for those that do not seek prompt treatment. A man recently diagnosed with prostate cancer may read such statistics with trepidation and fear. He might also be overwhelmed by the sheer volume of information available.

Doctors often push treatments they are familiar with and many men will accept the recommendation of a urologist without question or further research. Men diagnosed with prostate cancer often insist on getting immediate treatment. If you are one of them, be aware that you will likely question the wisdom of your decision on realizing the side effects of the surgery are permanent and not to your liking.

When the diagnosis is on an older patient, particularly one with significant other co-morbidities, all options should be explored with a goal is to avoid radical treatment where it would not prolong life.

Often a man will depend solely on his urologist for advice and treatment recommendations. Some may opt for a second opinion. Unscrupulous urologists may concur even if the cancer is not life-threatening. Prostat cancer is typically a slow growing cancer. Treating it in a hurry ofter benefits the practitioner much more tha it does the patient.

Since the addition of prostate specific antigen (PSA) testing to routin blood work for men over fifty, the risk for a man to be diagnosed with prostate cancer has increased substantially. Such a diagnosis usuall results in extreme duress and is often coupled with an emotional need for immediate treatment to "fix" or "remove" the cancer.

But since many cancers found via routine PSA testing are clinicall insignificant, aggressive treatment can be more damaging than helpful—especially to a man's quality of life. Recent news reports and guidelines confirm this.

Men diagnosed with prostate cancer are frequently scheduled for aggressive treatment within a few weeks (and sometimes within days of their diagnosis. Much of this is due to misinformation on the par of the patient, and a failure of the clinician to fully explain the risk benefit ratio. It is often easier to satisfy an emotional need for immediat treatment, than it is to explain to a panicky patient that his cancer ma never become life threatening or cause him any real problems.

This results in over-treatment of many cases of localized, low-risk non-aggressive prostate cancer. Unfortunately, prostate cancer treatmen has significant side effects, particularly on a man's quality of life. Without question, all treatment for prostate cancer—short of active surveillanc or watchful waiting—causes some degree of permanent sexua dysfunction and incontinence.

While some function may return after a few weeks or months, o sometimes years, it will never be the same as it was before treatmen Many men go into treatment without fully understanding this—only t have serious regrets later.

In today's society, we are conditioned to quickly treat all health problems that occur. Couple this mindset with the word cancer, and panic easily sets in. A doctor that feels immediate treatment is not mandatory may well find himself transferring patient records to someone else—even though a man with low-risk prostate cancer may be well advised to pursue a program of "watchful-waiting" or "active surveillance"—especially if he is 75 or older.

For many men and their clinicians though, "watchful waiting" simply means a repeat PSA test and biopsy every few months. During this time, the original conditions that caused the cancer to appear are not altered, and thus one is only waiting for the cancer to progress to a point where aggressive medical treatment is mandatory.

It is important for men to realize that there is an inherent wisdom in the body. There is very strong evidence that the right nutrients and herbal medication can help the body contain and possibly reverse the course of low-risk prostate cancer, potentially freeing the patient of the need to have aggressive treatment for years or for the rest of his life.

Many clinicians have limited knowledge of nutrition and herbal support and are reluctant to refer patients to naturopaths, herbalists, and/or nutritionists. In my opinion, they are doing their patients a great disservice.

Men with localized, low-risk, non-aggressive prostate cancer need to explore their options with both conventional and natural practitioners. They need to wake up to the enormous benefits and potential of natural health and nutrition and its role in preventing and reversing prostate problems.

A reputable and knowledgeable natural health practitioner can work side-by-side with a medical doctor resulting in better overall results for all patients, and particularly for men with prostate problems.

Keep in mind that all medical treatments for prostate cancer carry significant side effects, many of them sexual. Some of these side effects might be delayed for several years (especially those from radiation), but many are immediate. Virtually all of them are permanent. Think about never having a erection again.

Today, more urologists are becoming aware of the important role health supplements and nutrition can play in reducing the need for aggressive treatment of prostate cancer. These doctors are aware that watchful waiting along with a well-defined supplement program can be very valuable in helping their patients.

My recommendation, if you have been recently diagnosed with prostate cancer, is to learn as much as you can about the illness, and how you can fit it into your life plan without destroying yourself. Many intelligent men, when diagnosed with PC, research all kinds of conventional treatment options, and then choose a treatment.

Sometimes a natural option can reduce the need for treatment altogether. But, it does you little good if you never explore that option!

Prostatitis

P rostatitis is a common condition affecting men where the prostate becomes infected and inflamed. Its source can be either a bacterial or fungal infection, and it may be accompanied by severe pain, particularly in the area of the back and groin, inability to urinate, blood or pus in the urine, and a high fever.

Prostatitis is not cancer and studies show it does not cause or predispose a man to cancer. However, it is frequently associated with men that have Benign Prostate Hyperplasia (BPH). It is a common problem for men of all ages, and is most prevalent in middle-aged men between 35 and 55 years old. It is estimated to affect nearly half of all men at some point in their lives.

The male prostate tends to grow throughout life in most men. This continuing growth can increase the risk of prostatitis.

Medically it can appear as an acute bacterial infection and is treated with antibiotics. While antibiotics usually clear the active infection, they do not prevent it from reoccurring. When antibiotics do not relieve the issue quickly, the infection may be chronic or it may have a fungal source. Prostatitis that has a fungal source will typically become worse when antibiotics are used.

For some men, prostatitis can become chronic. Chronic bacterial prostatitis is a low-level bacterial infection of the prostate. It often presents with a minimum of symptoms and may linger for years. Medically, there is no known cure for the condition, although antibiotics used in the acute phase may help significantly. It does not appear to lead to more serious prostate disorders.

Most medical doctors are not knowledgeable or equipped to diagnose or treat fungal prostatitis. Treatment usually requires long-term (six months or longer) treatment with an oral anti-fungal agents. Prescription anti-fungal agents have some serious side effects, but herbal and nutritional agents are gentler.

Fungal prostatitis usually occurs in men that are prone to other fungal infections, so that can be a clue to diagnosis, especially if antibiotics fail. In my practice, I have had excellent success using properly formulated colloidal silver, a natural antifungal. Coconut oil and/or oregano oil also seem to work well. As with the prescription antifungal medication, the treatment is long-term.

Prostatitis Causes – Prostatitis can be caused by bacteria or fungi that embed themselves into the prostate gland. Their source can be either the urinary tract or the rectum. It can also result from various sexually transmitted diseases or, in the case of fungal prostatitis, from a fungal skin infection of the patient or frequent vaginal yeast infection of his sexual partner.

Acute bacterial prostatitis is often caused by common strains of bacteria such as; E. coli. The infection can be initiated when bacteria from anywhere leak into the prostate. It begins abruptly with high fever, chills, joint and muscle aches, and fatigue. It is typically diagnosed by patient symptoms, but blood and semen can also be tested for bacteria, white blood cells, or other signs of infection. If blood and semen do not indicate bacterial infection, the source may be physical (injury, etc.) or the prostatitis might be due to a fungal infection such as Candida.

Several medications are also known to cause or exacerbate prostate inflammation. Among these are:

- *Antihistamines typically used in cold medicines*
- *Nonsteroidal anti-inflammatory drugs (NSAIDs) like ibuprofen,*

naproxin, and ketoprofen, found in over the counter products
- *Prescription medications like Celebrex and Vioxx. (See caution note below)*
- *Some foods, particularly those in the pepper family may also trigger prostatitis*

Caution: Vioxx is no longer available in the US. However, the drug is till available in other countries under differing names. It was taken off he US market in 2004 after a study showed it caused increased risk of erious cardiovascular events. The manufacturer, Merck, has agreed to ay several billion dollars to settle thousands of lawsuits. If you have had rostatitis before, it is wise to avoid the above drugs. Any of them can rritate the prostate and cause more problems.

rostatitis is often associated with a urinary tract infection (UTI) and t can cause or exacerbate acute urinary retention or cause a sudden nability to urinate. Acute urinary retention can be quite painful and sually results in a visit to the emergency room for catheterization.

Prostatitis Symptoms: – Prostatitis is characterized by one or more of he following symptoms:

- *Painful, urgent, or frequent need to urinate.*
- *Burning sensation when urinating.*
- *Blood in the urine.*
- *Cloudy urine.*
- *Abdominal, rectal, groin or low back pain.*
- *Pain in the area just behind the scrotum or at the base of the penis.*
- *Pain during or after ejaculation.*
- *Fever, chills and/or malaise.*
- *Pus or other urethral discharge.*
- *Painful ejaculation.*

- *Sexual dysfunction. Typically ED or inability to ejaculate.*

Depending on the type and severity of the condition, some men ma
experience excruciating symptoms while others may simply have littl
to no bothersome symptoms. All types of prostatitis are treatable, bu
treatment approaches may be quite different, and very dependent on th
scope of the problem,. Many of the symptoms of prostatitis can als
be associated with urinary tract infections (UTIs) and the condition i
often accompanied by a coexisting UTI.

Prostatitis Treatment: – Conventional medical treatment fo
prostatitis is typically a fluoroquinolone antibiotic such as ciprofloxaci
(Cipro) or levofloxacin. According to a press release in Nov of 2018 from
the European Medicines Agency:

- *"These medicines can cause long-lasting, disabling and potentiall
  permanent side effects involving tendons, muscles, joints and the
  nervous system."*

There are two main ways prostatitis appears. The most serious is as a
acute bacterial infection in the prostate. It often appears associated with
UTI and is usually successfully treated with a short course of antibiotic
This is an emergency medical condition that should be treated promptl
by a qualified medical professional.

In many men, antibiotic treatment is all that is needed, but in som
recurrence occurs. When the condition recurs frequently, it is usuall
diagnosed as chronic bacterial prostatitis and treated with longer course
of antibiotics. This subacute prostate infection may also present wit
a variety of the above symptoms albeit at a lower level than the acut
infection, and is often characterized by recurrent urinary tract infection

When long-term courses of antibiotics do not resolve the conditio
completely, some practitioners will diagnose it as chronic pelvic pai

syndrome or inflammatory prostatitis. This diagnosis is quite common and the etiology is generally unknown. Many medical doctors have no idea how to treat it and sometimes recommend surgical removal of the prostate as a solution.

Caution: If a practitioner is recommending you have your prostate surgically removed due to prostatitis, my recommendation is to find another practitioner! There are no surgical treatments for prostatitis, but some recommend removal of the entire prostate gland (prostatectomy) as a solution.

Prostatectomy is major surgery involving the full range of associated surgical risks. Also, its long term side effects far outweigh the discomfort and danger of prostatitis. There are far simpler and less debilitating ways to resolve it, and a recommendation for surgery is, in my opinion, tantamount to overtreatment.

Men suffering from prostatitis often present at urology clinics for many years due to pelvic pain, urinary tract symptoms, and cloudy urine. While the condition is common, many practitioners are not well aware of it, especially when the etiology of the condition is fungal rather than bacterial. Suffering men are often treated for BPH and/or chronic bacterial prostatitis with little successful results.

Prostatitis that is non-bacterial should be investigated as possibly having a fungal source. Treatment requires long-term anti-fungal agents, either prescription or natural. (See Treating Fungal Prostatitis below.)

The antibiotic treatment is, of course, needed if the prostate infection is bacterial in nature. However, many practitioners have found that prostate infections and prostatitis are not always bacterial. Fungal prostatitis is also common in many men, especially those whose sexual partners are often subject to vaginal yeast infections.

Candidiasis is a fungal infection caused by the common yeast Candida albicans, a type of fungus. Candidiasis in the vagina is commonly referred to as a vaginal yeast infection. It is common in women and, if the fungus invades the prostate, it can result in fungal prostatitis.

A fungal infection of the prostate often results in many of the same symptoms as a bacterial infection. Fungal infections can be caused by microscopic fungi in the environment as well as sexual activity with a woman prone to, or with a vaginal yeast infection. Some men are also prone to fungal infections, usually of the skin.

Regardless of the source, once the fungus migrates and embeds itself into the prostate, it can cause prostatitis that mimics a bacterial infection. Some men, especially those that have compromised immune systems due to poor health or ongoing medical treatment, are more susceptible to fungal infections than healthy men, but it can strike anyone at any time.

Unfortunately, many practitioners dismiss fungal prostatitis infections as nonexistent simply because they are unfamiliar with them. Diagnosis can be established by urine cultures, symptom overview and a careful analysis. However, with a fungal infection, antibiotics are typically ineffective and may even make the condition worse by deteriorating beneficial bacteria that might be helping to keep the fungus from gaining total control.

Fungal prostatitis and UTIs affect mainly patients who have urinary tract obstruction accompanied with BPH or are immune-compromised by other medical treatments or diabetes, or both. They are common in men that are catheterized as a result of other medical treatments or urinary blockage.

- *A practitioner should suspect a fungal UTI in any patient with prostatitis who has clinical or laboratory findings consistent with UTI but with no bacterial findings.*

Fungal prostatitis can be treated using prescription antifungal medications, but natural antifungal treatment is more effective and has far less side effects. The list below shows some common natural antifungal agents:

- *Colloidal Silver – a therapeutic dose of colloidal silver appears to be most effective for both bacterial and fungal prostatitis. Typical dosing of a standard 25 ppm colloidal silver product is about 6-8 teaspoons/day, scaling down as the symptoms disappear and continuing for at least 1 to 2 months after symptoms resolve.*

- *Coconut oil – contains caprylic acid and other anti-microbial properties that are proven to kill yeasts, candida, and some bacteria. Studies have shown that it is more effective in treating candidiasis than many prescription drugs.*

- *Oregano oil – this herbal antifungal, while its taste is not very appetizing, is quite powerful. Oil of oregano is made from the leaves and shoots of the oregano plant (Origanum vulgare). It contains strong antifungals and antibacterial agents and research shows it can stop the growth of the various fungus species including Candida. It can be used to treat bacterial or fungal prostatitis by combining 3 to 4 drops with a teaspoon of coconut oil and taken internally two to three times daily*

- *Apple cider vinegar – this natural product is readily available and has been shown in studies to kill Candida fungus. It is more often used for fungal skin infections, but it is mild and can help control prostatitis if used long-term.*

- *Tea Tree oil – a well-known, topical treatment for various fungal and bacterial skin infections. However, it must be used internally with extreme caution. It should not be used internally except by a*

qualified practitioner and must be significantly diluted. Pure Tea
Tree oil can cause major irritation when used incorrectly. It is best
to leave its use to a skilled practitioner.

The prostate is an organ that contains many small capillaries and vessels.
When it is subject to infection, it is critical that the agent used to treat it
be applied on a long-term basis, so that it has a chance to reach infected
cells. A typical duration of treatment is at least three months for most
natural products. For some serious infections, treatment for up to a year
may be needed.

Note that disappearance of symptoms is not an indication that the
infection is eliminated. Some infections may appear to be eliminated in
as little as two weeks. Both fungal and bacterial infections of the prostate
can linger at a low, symptom-less level, only to flare up again if treatment
is terminated.

In cases where the man's sexual partner is subject to recurring vaginal
yeast infections, long-term treatment is necessary for both partners to
effect a cure.

Some medical doctors tend to minimize the impact of prostatitis on the
male population. Men that present with pelvic pain and inflammation
are often given a prescription for Cipro or a similar antibiotic without
further testing or analysis.

Non-bacterial prostatitis is not affected by antibiotics. And, if the
condition is due to a fungal overgrowth, an antibiotic might even
exacerbate it.

Many doctors are in denial about fungal sources of prostatitis. Reports
often dismiss it, but it appears that it is more widespread than generally
indicated. Men that are suffering, but have no confirmed diagnosis,
might find the medical consensus of opinion is wrong.

ortunately for many men, prostatitis is often a self-limiting condition that will sometimes resolve without the presence of an antibiotic or other medical intervention.

f a man is experiencing recurrent prostatitis, especially if there is no UTI present, a fungal source is likely. Sex with a partner that gets recurrent vaginal yeast infections could be a primary source and should be considered. Treatment as a couple might be needed to completely resolve the issue.

The primary purpose of the male prostate gland is to secrete fluid to lubricate and nourish ejaculated sperm. This secretion, combined with sperm cells produced by the testicles, makes up the bulk of the fluid released when a man ejaculates.

Men suffering with nonbacterial prostatitis, especially if they have a sparse sex life, should be encouraged to ejaculate regularly by masturbation. Studies show that prostate secretions can build up and cause prostatitis when left unreleased for long periods. Thus, normal and regular sexual activity can help decrease the incidence of prostate malfunction.

Prostatitis is a common condition, especially for older men. Urology clinics in the United States see about 2 million cases per year and more than 25 percent of men will receive a prostatitis diagnosis throughout their lifetime.

Autopsy studies find histologic presence of prostatitis in more than 50 percent of men examined. This alone indicates it is an under-diagnosed and under-treated condition in the United States. A man suffering from prostatitis, especially if the condition is constant, or reoccurs regularly, should seek medical help from a professional that is well versed in treating prostate issues and is aware of the latest research into this condition.

Testosterone

Testosterone is one member of a family of hormones called th sex-steroid hormones. Other members include progesteron dehydroepiandrosterone (DHEA), androstenediol, estriol, estron estradiol and dihydrotestosterone (DHT).

The androgens (testosterone, androstenedione, DHT) affect mostl male characteristics while the estrogens affect mainly femal characteristics. Others, like DHEA and progesterone are precursors use by the body to build other hormones. In the past progesterone an estradiol were thought to be strictly female hormones but recent researc indicates that the male prostate is rich in hormone receptors an sensitive to the effects of all hormones in this family, especiall progesterone.

The body normally converts some testosterone to DHT and estradio An excessively high testosterone level typically results in correspondingl high levels of DHT and estradiol. High values of these two hormone can exacerbate prostate enlargement, commonly known as benig prostate hyperplasia or BPH, and can also accelerate growth of a existing prostate tumor.

After reaching peak levels during his mid-to-late-20s, a man testosterone level begins a slow decline. From the age of about 35, drops by about 10 percent per decade for the rest of his life, accompanie by a slight increase in estrogen levels. In most men, this decreas contrary to what the "Low-T" ads say, does not cause significan problems.

Testosterone is an extremely important hormone both for developmen and maintenance of body functions both male and female. An extremel

42

low testosterone level can cause depression and is a risk factor for many chronic illnesses. Thus, it is prudent to measure your hormone levels now and then just to make certain everything is OK. This becomes more critical if you are having symptoms.

Hormones exist in two states: free (active) and bound (inactive). Only the free hormones attach to receptors on throughout the body to deliver their chemical message to the target organ. On average, approximately 97 to 98 percent of testosterone in a man's body is inactive, circulating in the blood bound to a blood protein called Sex Hormone Binding Globulin (SHBG). The two to three percent remaining portion (free value) is actually the only bio-available testosterone left to act on the body's receptors.

When testosterone is measured in blood, the bound and free values are usually combined into a single total value. In many cases, the ordering physician does not separately specify measurement of the free value, assuming that the body will convert the appropriate amount as needed. However, especially in older men, the conversion can be impaired due to an imbalance in other related hormones, illness, or medication. This is another reason why it is critically important to measure the full range of free values for at least five of the sex steroid hormones.

The range for free testosterone is typically calculated as a percentage of the total testosterone. But unfortunately, the reference range for total testosterone in blood (270-1100 ng/ml) is so wide that it becomes difficult to establish what is normal for a particular male. For example, an aging male with mid-range total testosterone might have extremely low conversion rate (less than one percent) to free testosterone.

If only the total is measured, (the usual case), his deficiency will go unnoticed, and he will continue to have symptoms. A healthy percentage of free testosterone is between two and three percent of the total value, but many men feel better when their free value is a little higher. Since saliva hormone testing measures only free hormone values, guess work and calculations are removed.

All of the sex steroid hormones are interdependent. An artificially high value in one can cause others to skew off the normal in either direction. A good example of this often occurs with male body-builders that use large amounts of androgen hormones to aid in muscle building. A substantial portion of these excess hormones is converted to the estrogens and DHT. This can result in unwanted breast growth (Gynecomastia), unwanted prostate growth (BPH) and testicular shrinking.

Yikes! – Testicular shrinkage! The human body is a smart organism, especially concerning hormones. It will always try to maintain an internal state of balance. The medical term for this is homeostasis. In the course of my career, I have had two clients that were body-builders and heavy users of artificial androgens. Both came to me because their testicles had shrunken to the size of raisins.

The testicles produce androgen hormones. If the body thinks it has an overabundance of androgens, it signals the testicles to shut down production. Like any other organ in the body, when there is nothing to do, atrophy sets in. So the testicles shrunk.

The first client was looking to me to tell him how to get his balls back. Unfortunately, I had nothing to tell him except to stop the anabolic steroids. I never saw the second fellow again, but I heard of his sudden death from a heart attack while he was working out and building his beautiful muscles. Both clients were in their mid-fifties.

This is why it is critically important to get hormone levels tested before attempting testosterone supplementation. Saliva testing is quick, private, and relatively inexpensive. Unlike blood testing, a saliva test measures only the critical free hormone levels. Most laboratories and many alternative health practitioners, recognizing the important interaction of hormones in the sex steroid family, recommend measuring free values of at least these five most critical hormones: progesterone, DHEA, testosterone, DHT and estradiol.

A practitioner can then review the results and if an imbalance indicates a need, supplementation can be instituted for one or more hormones. Thus, it is essential to test hormone levels before starting any replacement program, and to retest periodically to make sure the values are staying within the appropriate range. When only a single hormone like testosterone is tested, there is no knowledge of the status of the others, and supplementing based on this limited information is definitely a prescription for disaster!

In the past, much of the medical literature warned against testosterone supplementation, under the belief that it would increase the risk of prostate cancer. Recent research has shown this to be untrue. There is no evidence that restoring a man's testosterone level to its biological normal value will increase his risk of prostate cancer. In fact, many studies have determined the opposite. However, exceeding biological normal values can be very detrimental.

There are many different types of testosterone replacement therapies available. Most doctors use bi-weekly injections, but you can get transdermal patches, transdermal gels, implants embedded just under the skin that release the hormone over a long time period, and slow dissolving mouth patches.

However, most of these methods use synthetic testosterone, and they have unwanted side effects that may tend to cause problems.

The best way to use testosterone therapy is to use a bio-identical testosterone cream that is either prepackaged (Testim, Androgel) or mixed to your doctor's prescription by a compounding pharmacy. The latter may be considerably less expensive. One of the advantages of the compounded cream is that the prescribing doctor can make minor adjustments to his dosage depending on his response. In addition, the patient himself can make adjustments to his dosage quite easily by using more or less of the cream.

Testosterone Supplementation: – As a man passes the age of fifty he often finds himself encountering problems he never knew existed in his youth. Suddenly, he may find he is unable to perform sexually at the same level as before, and in some cases, he may be experiencing some degree of erectile dysfunction. In our society today, advertisements about low testosterone, AKA low-T, bombard us daily. Thus, when problems arise, most men—and their doctors—often start thinking about testosterone levels before anything else.

A subsequent visit to a doctor typically results in blood tests that include a testosterone level, as well as a host of other tests. If the man's testosterone measurement comes back below the normal range, his doctor may simply write a prescription for testosterone supplementation or an erectile dysfunction drug or both. The ED drug might help If his problem is erectile dysfunction, but is of little help for the myriad of other sexual issues.

When the prescription doesn't help, he might be told "Well, you're getting older. You just have to accept that you cannot perform like before." Unfortunately, some men accept this, and go through the rest of their lives suffering with problems that might be easily remedied had they—or their doctors—been willing to spend the time to look deeper.

Some men strongly feel the effects of a cumulative decline in testosterone levels and experience significant symptoms, while others barely notice it. For men that acutely feel the effects, Restoring testosterone to its biological norm can be very rewarding.

Testosterone supplementation is indeed needed for many older men to bring levels back to a biological normal value. The keywords here are biological normal. Media advertising makes it seem like it testosterone supplementation is a harmless way to increase stamina, energy and sexual performance for any man. Nothing could be further from the truth.

Excess testosterone—beyond a biological normal value—is linked to many serious medical conditions, most notably heart attack and stroke. With hormones, enough is good, but more is definitely counterproductive and can be damaging.

Past incorrect beliefs that testosterone replacement therapy causes prostate cancer left many medical practitioners reluctant to prescribe it. The latest scientific research shows that a healthy man does not increase disease risks by raising his testosterone level to the normal biological range for his age.

Renowned medical oncologist and prostate cancer researcher and survivor, Dr. Charles "Snuffy" Myers, has stated, "There is absolutely no hint that testosterone at high levels correlates with prostate cancer." He founded the American Institute for Diseases of the Prostate, near Charlottesville, Virginia.

Natural bioidentical testosterone cream labeled USP, for United States Pharmacopeia standard, is available at compounding pharmacies. Bioidentical means that a substance has the same chemical form as that produced by the human body.

Other forms of testosterone therapy, including biweekly injections, skin patches and pills typically employ synthetic chemicals that are similar, but not identical, to natural testosterone. Thus, such products are not completely recognizable by the body.

Several years ago, bestselling author and hormone balancing expert Dr. John R. Lee published his startling conclusion that synthetic hormones

can cause serious side effects, including an increased risk of stroke, cance
and liver damage. His findings were subsequently confirmed by th
Women's Health Initiative study. Injections, skin patches and pill
subject the body to unnatural fluctuations in testosterone and estroger
In contrast, skin creams can permit precise periodic dosing.

Remember that hormones are powerful and a little can go a long wa
Beyond bringing a man's hormone levels back to biological norma
more is not better and can reverse benefits.

Contrary to popular belief and media dogma, ED is typically not th
result of a low total testosterone level, but a low free testosterone leve
may cause a man to experience of loss of libido or nocturnal erections.

Urinary Retention

Urinary retention is a very common side effect of aging men that also have benign prostate hypertrophy (BPH). It occurs when a man cannot fully empty his urinary bladder and retains urine within the bladder. Another, less common cause for the condition is a weak bladder muscle unable to contract strongly enough to empty the bladder. In this chapter, I refer to only the type of retention caused by BPH.

The urinary bladder, located in the lower abdomen just below the navel, is very similar to a balloon. Its purpose is to expand and collect urine output from the kidneys and contract on urination as it empties. Urinary retention occurs when the bladder cannot empty completely. When this happens the condition can be either acute, where urination is suddenly impossible, or chronic, where the person cannot empty the bladder completely.

Chronic urinary retention can cause serious kidney damage over time. It is insidious and generally causes few symptoms except a need to urinate more often than prior years. Older men tend to notice it by the need to use the bathroom more frequently. It is frequently overlooked by many men as just normal part of aging until the symptoms become serious enough for him to consult a doctor. Often, the wake-up call is an urgent trip to the ER due to an inability to urinate at 3am.

For many men, aging results in an enlargement of the prostate gland, but while aging is surely a risk for BPH, hormone imbalances, poor diet, and especially excess estrogen levels can also cause it. A man suffering from BPH is well advised to have a home salivary hormone test that measures several of his sex steroid hormones before starting any medical or natural treatment to resolve BPH.

With BPH, a man typically suffers a decrease in urinary flow as his growing prostate compresses and narrows the tube that passes urine from his urinary bladder (the urethra). As long as the decreased flow is not significant, it is usually not a problem. However, when the blockage seriously affects the flow of urine, it causes urine to accumulate in the bladder beyond the normal level of 50 to 100 ml.

The accumulated urine in the bladder can cause back pressure into the man's kidneys. This back pressure can damage the kidneys since they have no means to force the urine through the tubes (ureters) that lead to the bladder. If the bladder is somewhat full, the urine backs up into the kidneys and causes damage to its delicate passages..

Urinary retention in older men is almost always caused by an enlarged prostate gland (BPH). When a man has BPH, any disturbance that causes a temporary swelling or inflammation of the prostate can result in a temporary inability to urinate. This *acute* urinary retention is a situation requiring immediate treatment to avoid kidney damage. It can occur suddenly without an obvious trigger or can be due to physical activity or a prostate infection (See prostatitis above).

Acute urinary retention typically occurs to a man during the night time hours, and he usually winds up in the emergency room, painfully waiting for someone to catheterize him to alleviate the over-pressure situation in his bladder. A tube, (called a Foley catheter) is typically inserted through his penis and into his bladder in the ER setting, immediately relieving the acute stress on the kidneys and the bladder.

When the man is usually released from the ER, with a catheter and a collection bag in place, and told to make a follow-up appointment with a urologist.

A Foley catheter is typically used in the hospital or urologist environment. It consists of a pair of thin, plastic tubes inserted through the penile urethra into the bladder. A small balloon at the bladder end of one of the tubes is inflated with sterile water after the catheter is threaded into the bladder. This balloon, when inflated, keeps the catheter from inadvertently slipping out.

The second tube is the conduit used to transport urine out of the bladder and into a plastic collection bag, usually secured to the the patients leg. Thus, a Foley catheter can be left in place for a period of time. However, the longer it is in place, the higher the risk of a bladder infection.

For many men, this is where a downward roller coaster slide begins. The lucky guy keeps the catheter in for a few days to a week or so, then goes to the urologist, gets it removed and is able to urinate normally again. The unlucky guy gets the catheter removed, still can't urinate, and the catheter is replaced the same day or after a short trial period of a few hours.

What many guys don't realize is that even if you are in the unlucky group, urinary function will likely return to normal, it just may take a little longer. However, it is at this time that the man is most vulnerable to falling towards that downward slide mentioned above.

Caution: An unscrupulous doctor might insist that the problem can be only be fixed by a procedure called a Trans-Urethral-Prostatectomy (TURP), and that the procedure should be done immediately.

A TURP removes part of the prostate gland blocking the urethra through an instrument passed through the penis. The instrument holds a cutting tool (knife or laser), a viewing instrument (cystoscope) with an associate light (and possibly a camera), so the surgeon can view the internal area. Excess prostate tissue is removed through the tube and discarded. Hopefully, after the man heals, his urinary stream will be much improved.

While a TURP may indeed be needed for some men. It is wise to wait a little while after an acute event and seek some natural support for the probelm.

Above I mentioned the "downward roller coaster slide." This is the point at which the unwary guy gets talked into having a TURP procedure long before he has investigated or exhausted other, more simple or natural techniques. A TURP is a surgical procedure. While it is relatively minor, it still carries many of the same risks as other surgical procedures. In addition, it also has unwanted side effects. If the condition can be resolved naturally with herbal remedies or lifestyle factors, the end result can be much more rewarding.

Chronic urinary retention caused by BPH is typically treated using prescription drugs like Flomax or natural remedies that contain combinations of saw palmetto and pygeum. While Flomax is well-tested for relieving urinary retention, it is also known to have negative sexual side effects. These include abnormal ejaculation, inability to ejaculate, decreased ejaculate and retrograde ejaculation (little or no semen expelled from the penis on orgasm). Studies have also noted that some men have new onset ED after a TURP procedure.

A natural substitute for Flomax is the herbs above along with a mixture of flower pollen from various grass types. I have had good success in my practice using an herb named Swedish Flower Pollen. It has similar characteristics as Flomax, but virtually no side effects.

Unfortunately, herbal products are at the mercy of the manufacturer. While they may contain the right ingredients, they may not contain a therapeutic dose, may be inefficiently or improperly extracted, or may contain the wrong form of the herb. Selecting a quality herbal product usually means consulting an natural health expert or naturopath with extensive experience and knowledge that will usually know the most well-known and regarded sources.

Many products on the market (usually tagged with words like male support or male enhancement) contain little of the active ingredients that actually support a healthy prostate. Many of these products are geared to improve sexual stamina or libido and may have a deleterious effect on proper prostate functioning.

If you are also having sexual difficulties, it is wise to consider healing your prostate as your first priority. Improving prostate and overall health may restore poor sexual function. Stay away from products containing herbs touted to increase libido such as TongCat Ali, Yohimbe, Tribulus and Maca unless your prostate is already healthy and you are strictly looking to improve libido and sexual performance. These herbs are valuable in that sense, and they often find their way into many over-the-counter male formulas, but they do little to enhance overall prostate health.

Hormone levels also play a strong role in the development of BPH and subsequent urinary retention. It is well known that excess estrogen levels can trigger prostate growth, BPH and even prostate cancer. A salivary hormone test is simply done in the privacy of your home and measures both androgen and estrogen levels. It can help your provider isolate a hormonal imbalance that can then be corrected naturally with either diet modifications or bio-identical hormones.

If all else fails, you may need to use a catheter for a while your prostate returns to some semblance of normal. There are generally three types of catheters.

- An in-dwelling or Foley catheter which is typically used in a hospital or urologist setting in response to an acute urinary blockage. It can be put in place for a few days or several weeks and is connected to a collection bag.
- A condom catheter, which is typically used for temporary incontinence. It has a condom-like tip that adheres to the tip of the penis and is also connected to a collection bag.

- A simple self-catheter can be used while the prostate is healing after an acute incident, or used by older men that do not want to risk TURP surgery. This type of catheter is used as needed and is removed after draining the bladder of urine. It can be used several times per day and men that have disturbed sleep because of frequent nighttime urination often self-catheterize at bedtime for a better night's sleep.

The bottom line is that there are many ways to alleviate the urinar retention issues associated with BPH. The best way is to resolve o improve the BPH condition. Any man that has such issues would b wise to see a natural health professional while these issues are just mildl annoying before he finds himself in a medical emergency situatior rushing to the ER at 3 a.m., with a painfully full urinary bladder.

Conclusion

———

As I mentioned above, a healthy lifestyle and diet can go a long way to helping you avoid many of the pitfalls of aging. Good health (and good erections) depend on blood circulation. Anything that impairs it increases risks: smoking, excess alcohol consumption, diabetes, obesity, high cholesterol or blood pressure, heart disease, and a sedentary lifestyle.

Many of the pitfalls of aging that cause problems are due to the excess media advertising for pharmaceutical agents. Each carrying the ubiquitous statement to "ask your doctor if *XX* is right for you."

With this thought ingrained in them, many people wind up with a prescription drug list a mile long. And, a doctor that refuses to prescribe a drug the patient believes will help him will likely lose a patient, which puts the doctor in a financial bind. Note that most pharmaceutical drugs do not cure an illness, they simply cover up its symptoms.

Caution: – Every pharmaceutical drug has side effects. Some may be very minimal and some can be life-threatening. Question your provider and/or do your own research.

If you do your own drug research, it is best to stay clear of the pharmaceutical manufacturers site except for the basic information. They are often very vague about the side effects of their drugs. Peer-to-peer sites for a drug are sometimes useful, but they need to be used intelligently. Some folks post and complain about everything. Generally, if a problem gets recurrent posts of essentially the same problem on a peer-to-peer site you can assume it is likely a real issue.

Drugs used to treat various prostate and as well as other health problems frequently alter sexual performance in a negative way. Some drugs are known to inhibit erections, others can effect orgasms. Every drug you are on should be researched (preferably by you), so that you know what its side effects might be. You may want to do something like a "Risk/ Reward" analysis to determine whether this drug is right for you. You doctor should be doing this, but....

If you have doubts, pin your doctor down and get your doubts resolved toyour satisfaction. If your doctor refuses to talk to you about your drugs in detail, find another doctor.

A true case study: An 84 YO female relative was rushed by ambulance to the hospital with life threatening low blood pressure. She was, at the time, on 28 different prescription medications. Her condition was traced back to several drugs that combined to cause her potassium levels to drop severely. Her doctor should have been aware of this, but never checked for it.

According to the American Association of Consultant Pharmacists, seniors over 80 YO fill an average of 18 prescriptions per year. Seniors often visit multiple doctors. In the above case, the lady had visited several different doctors, each one adding to her list of drugs without any real analysis of the drugs already on the list from other providers.

The doctors in the case above should have been more careful to analyze the drugs the lady was taking. However, they did not and it nearly cost her her life.

Caution:—The medical term that applies to the above is *Iatrogenic*. It indicates a condition or illness caused by the activity of a physician, therapy, or medication.

While most medical offices collect a list of drugs a patient is on, it is rare that this list is evaluated to see if the drugs on it are appropriate for the patients condition. A recent Institute of Medicine report estimated 230,000 to 284,000 iatrogenic deaths annually.

The Bottom Line

——

You and only you are responsible for your health an your treatment. Far too many people treat their doctors as if they are all-knowing deities. While most medical doctors are both qualified and conscientious, it is unrealistic to expect one you see for a few minutes, perhaps every six months or so, to know or solve all of your problems.

Unfortunately, this is often the case. People expect their doctors to be able to resolve all of their problems, and when this is not forthcoming, they refuse to take responsibility for their health.

I twenty plus years of practice, I have seen many guys and gals with typical aging problems that can not even readily describe their problem to me. Men in particular, are real masters of this, especially when it comes to sexual problems.

I often see men that cannot even refer to their penis effectively. I have heard it called a Johnson, Pole, Staff, Woodie and numerous other terms. Sometimes, their embarrassment misleads me to wrong conclusions.

In today's society, people tend to handle their overall health and healthcare in three different ways. First, there are those that have a firmly entrenched belief that they can get all of their needed vitamins, minerals and nutrients from the food they eat, even if their diet is very poor. The second group consists of those who are convinced that science and pharmaceuticals present an easily available cure for everything that bothers them. Finally, group three consists of people that carefully watch their health, eat well, research any problems they may encounter, and take supplements to help maintain good health.

The first two groups typically spend a lot of time in doctor's waiting rooms, hoping for a miracle procedure or drug that will make them well and feel better. The last group become active partners with their doctors, keep an open relationship, and generally get the most out of every doctor visit.

Again, only you are responsible for your health and your treatment. If you are unable or unwilling to describe your problem in exact detail to your doctor, then you cannot expect your doctor to help you fix it effectively.

Don't miss out!

Visit the website below and you can sign up to receive emails whenever James Occhiogrosso publishes a new book. There's no charge and no obligation.

https://books2read.com/r/B-A-AOZG-VVZBB

BOOKS 2 READ

Connecting independent readers to independent writers.

Also by James Occhiogrosso

Solutions for Erectile Dysfunction
Your Prostate, Your Libido, Your Life
Dr. Jim's Guide to the Aging Male Body

Watch for more at www.prostatehealthnaturally.com/index.html.

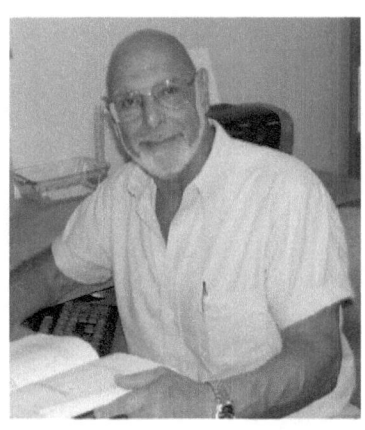

About the Author

James Occhiogrosso, N.D. is a Natural Health Practitioner specializing in male and female health issues and author of "Your Prostate, Your Libido, Your Life" and "Solutions for Erectile Dysfunction." He maintains an active practice helping both men and women overcome hormonal and sexual issues associated with aging, including loss of libido, erectile dysfunction and menopausal issues, and often acts as an advisor for men with prostate cancer whose doctors recommend a "watchful waiting" approach. Salivary home hormone test kits as well as bio-identical hormone creams are available at his website

He lives with his wife of nearly 40 years in Southwest Florida, USA